BEAUTIFUL COCKTAILS

100 cocktails that you will love.

A variety of colors and tastes
of the best cocktails.

The Beverage Kitchen

TABLE OF CONTENT

Green Mamba Long Drink

Green sky

Grasshopper

Green Gin Cocktail

Green meadow

Tropical green

Southern Comfort

Rosato Mio

Spain

Passion fruit squirt

Tequila Sunrise

Aperol-Gin Sour

Irish colada

Ipanema Rum

Zombie

Mai Tai

Aperol injection

Arabic Sun

Raspberry - Passion Fruit - Cocktail

Vitamin gel

Italian Gipsy

enchilada cooler

Spidu

Strong Aperol

Orange Dust

Watermelon daiquiri

Cream cocktail

Advocaat with sparkling wine and grenadine

Strawberry Kiss

Tinto de Verano

Strawberry colada

Ramazzotti Rosato Duo

Strawberry Daiquiri

9 Pin Gin

May Tai Mix

Lemonades Liqueur

Aperol spray

Pomegranate - Sparkling wine

Strawberry Mojito

Tinto de Verano

Tocco Rosso

Aperol Lemon Spray

Strawberry - sparkling wine

Ouzo Special

Beer cocktail with ginger ale

Fragolino

Strawberry - Lime

Bicicletta - Campari

Raspberry Mojito

Rhubarb Wine

Campari-O

Spritz with elderberry and basil

Cocktail Ruby

bloody caipirinha

gin fizz

Spray limoncello

Codka

BATIDA DE COCO

Color of the cocktail: Yellow
Servings: 1

ingredients
3 cl cachaça
4 cl pineapple juice
1 cl cream
2 cl Batida de Coco

Preparation
Prepare ingredients in an electric mixer on crushed ice. Pour into a long drink glass filled with ice.

SWEET PUNCH

Color of the cocktail: Yellow
Servings: 1

ingredients
4 cl rum, brown
6 cl passion fruit juice
6 cl ginger ale
2 cl water
Ice cube

Preparation
Pour everything into a glass and add the ice. You can vary the sweetness depending on how much water you add.

PONCHA

Color of the cocktail: Yellow
Servings: 1

ingredients
2 cl orange juice
1 cl lemon juice
2 cl honey
2 cl cachaça
Lemon juice
Sugar

Preparation
Dip the rim of the glass in lemon juice and then in the sugar.
Put all the ingredients into the glass and stir vigorously
until the honey has dissolved. In Madeira, the stirring is
done in a large vessel with a unique, wooden stick.

VIRGIN MARALIM

Color of the cocktail: Yellow
Servings: 1

ingredients
Ice cube
2 cl passion fruit syrup
3 cl vodka
½ Passion fruit
½ Lime
100 ml apple juice
20 ml of water

Preparation
Cut a slice from half of the washed lime and cut the rest into fingertip-sized pieces. Fill a cocktail glass 3/4 full with ice and moisten it with the passion fruit syrup. Sprinkle the passion fruit and the lime pieces on top and fill up with the apple juice and water until just under the rim. Finally stir the cocktail and make it pretty with the slice of lime.

IRISH MULE

Color of the cocktail: Yellow
Servings: 1

ingredients
Ice cube
50 ml of whiskey
17 ml of lime juice
17 ml lime syrup
200 ml ginger ale
1 lime slices

Preparation
Fill a large long drink glass with ice, add whiskey, juice,
syrup,half-filled and ginger ale and garnish with a slice of lime.

BAHAMA MOM

Color of the cocktail: Yellow-Beige
Servings: 1

ingredients
15 ml of coconut rum
15 ml rum, brown
15 ml coffee liqueur
15 ml rum, white
Ice cube
Pineapple juice
1 piece of pineapple

Preparation
Put Malibu, Kahlua, brown and white rum in a shaker and shake vigorously. Pour into a long drink glass half filled with crushed ice. Fill up with pineapple juice. Garnish with a thin slice of pineapple.

LEMON GINGER LEMONADE

Color of the cocktail: yellow-green
Servings: 4

ingredients
80 g sugar, brown
45 g ginger root
8 cl rum, white
1 large lemon
1 liter of water
Water, carbonated

Preparation
Put the brown sugar into a blender jug and work it into
icing sugar with a few turns. Cut the ginger and lemon
(complete with peel) into large cubes and add both to the
sugar in the blender. Puree until a thick paste is formed.
Then add the still water and mix again vigorously. Then
pour into a bottle through a fine sieve. Put in a cool place.

Pour the chilled lemonade and rum into a glass and
top up with sparkling mineral water as desired. If
necessary, add a few ice cubes and lemon slices.

COCKTAIL FRUIT CUP

Color of the cocktail: yellow-green
Servings: 1

ingredients
10 cl passion fruit juice
3 cl rum (white)
6 cl pineapple juice
6 cl lemon juice
4 cl orange juice
1 teaspoon Blue Curaçao
Ice cube

Preparation
Shake the juices and rum with some ice cubes in a shaker
for 1 minute, then strain into glasses with ice.

Drizzle a teaspoon of Blue Curaçao over it and
serve decorated as desired with fruit.

CAIPIRINHA GIN

Color of the cocktail: yellow-orange
Servings: 1

ingredients
½ Lime
6 cl ginger ale
4 cl gin
2 tsp sugar, brown
Passion fruit juice
Ice cube

Preparation
Cut half the lime into small pieces. Mix with the brown
sugar and crush it. Then add the ginger ale, gin, and
ice cubes and pour on the passion fruit juice.

WINE TONIC

Color of the cocktail: yellow-white
Servings: 4

ingredients
400 ml wine, white, dry
400 ml tonic water
8 leaves mint
4 slices of lemon
Ice cube

Preparation

Place 2 leaves of fresh mint and half a slice of lemon in each glass, add 100 ml of dry white port and some ice cubes and top up with 100 ml of tonic water.

GREEN ALMOND

Color of the cocktail: Green
Servings: 1

ingredients
2 cl Amaretto
2 cl Blue Curaçao
4 cl orange juice
2 cl cream
4 ice cubes

Preparation
Measure the ingredients, mix, and enjoy ice-cold.

RUM DE COCO

Color of the cocktail: Green
Servings: 2

ingredients
20 cl pineapple juice
8 cl Batida de Coco
5 cl coconut milk
4 cl rum, white
4 cl Blue Curaçao
2 cl lemon juice
6 ice cubes

Preparation
Place all ingredients (well chilled) together in a blender jug and foam for about 1 minute at the highest setting.

GREEN TEA FIZZ

Color of the cocktail: Green
Servings: 1

ingredients
150 ml tea, green
1 tsp honey
3 cl gin
Ice cube
100 ml tonic water
1 dash of lemon juice

Preparation
Brew 1 bag of green tea with 150 ml of water, sweeten with honey, and let cool. Put the tea into a long drink glass, add ice cubes, gin. Add tonic water and refine it with a dash of lemon.

BOLSWHEAT

Color of the cocktail: Green
Servings: 1

ingredients
500 ml of wheat beer
1 part Blue Curaçao
1 part orange juice

Preparation
Take a glass of wheat beer (0.5 l), fill it to one third
with Blue Curacao, to another third with orange juice,
and finally add one-third light wheat beer.

SOLERO

Color of the cocktail: Green
Servings: 1

ingredients
8 cl passion fruit juice
8 cl mango juice
2 cl vanilla syrup
2 cl rum
2 cl cream
Ice

Preparation
Fill ice cubes and all ingredients into a shaker and shake vigorously. Use 2-4 cl rum depending on the strength.

Pour into a chilled long drink glass. Decorate as desired.

ROMULAN

Color of the cocktail: Green
Servings: 1

ingredients
1 cl rum
1 cl melon liqueur
2 cl Amaretto
2 cl wormwood, sweet
2 cl Blue Curaçao
6 cl vodka

Preparation
Shake all ingredients together thoroughly.
Pour into a glass and serve.

WALDMEISTER BEER

Color of the cocktail: Green
Servings: 1

ingredients
2 tablespoons woodruff syrup
1 tsp lemon juice
1 bottle of wheat beer

Preparation
Put 2 tablespoons of syrup and 1 teaspoon of lemon
juice into each Berliner Weisse glass, fill up with 1
bottle of wheat beer and serve with a straw.

GREEN MAMBA LONG DRINK

Color of the cocktail: Green
Servings: 1

ingredients
2 cl lemon juice
10 cl passion fruit juice
4 cl liqueur 43
2 cl Blue Curaçao
2 cl cream
1 mint leaf
Ice cube

Preparation
Shake all ingredients well with 6-8 ice cubes in a shaker. Strain into a long drink glass on a few ice cubes. Garnish with a mint leaf.

GREEN SKY

Color of the cocktail: Green
Servings: 2

ingredients
6 cl Triple Sec
5 cl vodka
4 cl Blue Curaçao
1 orange
1 lime
200 ml tonic water
Ice cube

Preparation
Squeeze the orange and lime, pour the juice with Triple Sec, Blue
Curacao, vodka, and 3 ice cubes into a shaker and shake well.

Fill 2 long drink glasses up to half with ice cubes
and tonic water. Pour the canceled shaker contents
over the back of a spoon to form a layer.

GRASSHOPPER

Color of the cocktail: Green
Servings: 1

ingredients
2 cl cream
2 cl chocolate liqueur, brown
2 cl peppermint liqueur, green
Ice cube

Preparation
Shake the ingredients well on several ice cubes in
a shaker, pour into the glass, and enjoy.

GREEN GIN COCKTAIL

Color of the cocktail: Green
Servings: 1

ingredients
6 cl gin
2 cl lemon juice
2 cl sugar syrup
3 slices of cucumber
1 sprig of mint
1 shot of apple juice
Ice cube

Preparation
Place the gin with the ice cubes, lemon juice, sugar syrup, cucumber slices, and mint in a shaker and shake vigorously. Pour through a sieve into a glass with fresh ice cubes and add a dash of apple juice (until the glass is full).

GREEN MEADOW

Color of the cocktail: Green
Servings: 1

ingredients
4 cl Blue Curaçao
4 cl vodka
16 cl orange juice
Ice cube

Preparation
First, pour Curacao into the glass, fill up with the orange juice. Add ice cubes as desired.

TROPICAL GREEN

Color of the cocktail: Green
Servings: 1

ingredients
2 cl Batida de Coco
2 cl Blue Curaçao
10 cl pineapple juice

Preparation
Just mix everything with a little crushed ice.,

SOUTHERN COMFORT

Color of the cocktail: green-blue
Servings: 1

ingredients
50 ml liqueur, Southern Comfort
50 ml of lemon juice
100 ml of cola
Ice cube

Preparation
First, mix lemon juice with the Southern Comfort.
Pour this into a long drink glass and top it up with
cola. A few ice cubes in and that's it.

ROSATO MIO

Color of the cocktail: Light red
Servings: 1

ingredients
5 cl Ramazzotti
10 cl Prosecco
Ice cube
Basil

Preparation
Pour Ramazzotti Aperitivo Rosato and Prosecco into a wine glass. Add the ice cubes. Garnish the drink with some basil leaves.

SPAIN

Color of the cocktail: Orange
Servings: 1

ingredients
3 cl liqueur 43
2 cl vodka
2 cl cream
10 cl passion fruit juice
1 cl Grenadine

Preparation
Shake all ingredients except the grenadine in a shaker with ice cubes and strain into a long drink glass. Then pour the grenadine over it.

PASSION FRUIT SQUIRT

Color of the cocktail: Orange
Servings: 1

ingredients
4 cl Aperol
8 cl Passionfruit nectar
1 dash of lime juice
4 cl Prosecco
1 shot of mineral water
Ice cube

Preparation
Put the ice cubes in the glass. Add the Aperol, lime juice, and passion fruit nectar and top up with prosecco and mineral water.

Serve garnished with strawberries, blackberries or lemon slices as desired.

TEQUILA SUNRISE

Color of the cocktail: Orange
Servings: 1

ingredients
4 cl Tequila, white
15 cl orange juice
1 cl Grenadine
Ice

Preparation
Put the ice cubes into a long drink glass, pour the tequila
into it and top up with the orange juice. Add
the grenadine and stir a little.

APEROL-GIN SOUR

Color of the cocktail: Orange
Servings: 1

ingredients
4 cl Aperol
4 cl gin
2 cl lemon juice
2 teaspoons sugar
4 ice cubes

Preparation
Put all ingredients into a whiskey cup and stir.

IRISH COLADA

Color of the cocktail: Orange
Servings: 1

ingredients
4 cl cream liqueur
2 cl coconut rum
1 cl Grenadine
½ cl lime juice
10 cl pineapple juice

Preparation
Mix in a household blender and serve on ice.

IPANEMA RUM

Color of the cocktail: Orange
Servings: 1

ingredients
½ Lime
2 cl white rum
2 tablespoons cane sugar
60 ml passion fruit juice
60 ml ginger ale
Ice cube

Preparation
Cut half the lime into four pieces and put it into
the glass, sprinkle the cane sugar over it, and
crush it thoroughly with the pestle.

Add the passion fruit juice, rum, for and ginger ale and stir
the mixture with a straw to dissolve the limes and sugar.
Then fill a good portion of ice cubes into the glass.

ZOMBIE

Color of the cocktail: Orange
Servings: 1

ingredients
2 cl rum, white
2 cl rum, brown
1 cl apricot brandy
5 cl pineapple juice
2 cl lime juice
2 cl rum, 75%
1 slice orange
1 sprig of mint
1 cocktail cherry

Preparation
Shake ingredients except the 75% rum in a shaker with
ice and fill into the long drink glass with ice cubes.
Put the decoration on the sticker over the
glass, put mint in the glass.
Add 75% rum to the glass before serving.

MAI TAI

Color of the cocktail: Orange
Servings: 1

ingredients
4 cl rum, white
2 cl Amaretto
2 cl Triple Sec
2 cl rum, brown
100 ml of orange juice
100 ml pineapple juice
Grenadine
Ice cube

Preparation
Shake alcohol and juices with ice in a shaker vigorously, pour
into a long drink glass, with ice cubes, pour - carefully dribble
some grenadine on the ice cubes - put an orange slice and a
cocktail cherry on a sticker and serve with a long straw.

APEROL INJECTION

Color of the cocktail: Orange
Servings: 1

ingredients
4 cl Aperol
2 cl lemon juice
2 cl orange juice
Sparkling wine
Sparkling mineral water
Ice cube
Orange

Preparation
Put the ice cubes into a large cocktail or red wine glass.
Pour Aperol, lemon, and orange juice on the ice cubes.

Then fill up the glass with champagne. If you don't like
it quite so strong, you can also mix mineral water and
sparkling wine in equal parts. Serve with a straw.

ARABIC SUN

Color of the cocktail: Orange
Servings: 1

ingredients
15 cl orange juice
5 cl Triple Sec
1 cl pomegranate syrup
1 slice orange

Preparation
Fill a regular glass (not a flat glass) with Triple Sec and orange juice, then add the pomegranate syrup. Leave to stand for a few minutes so that the syrup can settle at the bottom. Garnish with an orange slice.

RASPBERRY - PASSION FRUIT - COCKTAIL

Color of the cocktail: Orange
Servings: 1

ingredients
100 ml passion fruit juice
2 cl rum
20 ml raspberry syrup
50 ml of milk
1 orange slice
Ice cube

Preparation
Put all ingredients together with some ice
in a shaker and shake vigorously.
Put some ice cubes in a long drink glass and pour the cocktail
over it. Decorate with a slice of orange and serve immediately.

VITAMIN GEL

Color of the cocktail: Orange
Servings: 1

ingredients
150 ml multivitamin juice
2 scoops of vanilla ice cream
50 ml sparkling wine
1 shot of raspberry syrup
1 orange slice
Water
Sugar

Preparation
Melt 1 scoop of vanilla ice cream into sauce. Place glass with the upper rim in water and then in sugar so that a sugar rim is formed. Then add 150 ml of multivitamin juice to the glass, then pour the champagne on top. Pour the vanilla sauce over the sparkling wine. Do not stir! Carefully add the second scoop of vanilla ice cream to the cocktail. Now put an orange slice on the rim of the glass.

ITALIAN GIPSY

Color of the cocktail: Orange
Servings: 1

ingredients
4 cl Aperol
4 cl orange juice
Champagne, dry, ice-cold
2 ice cubes
1 strawberry,

Preparation
Place two ice cubes in a stem glass. Pour the Aperol and juice over them. Top up with champagne and stir gently.

Make a slight lateral incision in the strawberry and stick it to the edge of the glass.

ENCHILADA COOLER

Color of the cocktail: Orange
Servings: 1

ingredients
2 cl lemon juice
2 cl lime juice
1 cl Grenadine
3 cl rum, white
3 cl Triple Sec
2 cl cherry brandy
2 cl apricot brandy
3 cl pineapple juice
3 cl orange juice
¼ Lime
Ice cube

Preparation
For the cocktail you need huge glasses. The ingredients
are matched to cocktail glasses with 550 ml content.

First, fill the glasses halfway, possibly a little higher, but not more
than 2/3, with ice cubes. Then pour the liquid ingredients in the
order mentioned above, from lemon juice to passion fruit juice,
over them. This sequence should be followed because of the
desired color gradient. The passion fruit juice is added at the end.

Finally, squeeze the lime pieces slightly above the glass
and then simply throw the pieces into the glass. The limes
must be washed thoroughly and hot beforehand. Otherwise,
the greasy coating will give off a very bitter taste.

SPIDU

Color of the cocktail: Orange
Servings: 1

ingredients
50 cl sparkling wine
50 cl lemonade
1 ice cube
1 mint leaf

Preparation
Put the sparkling wine and juice, well chilled in a champagne glass and serve with an ice cube and a mint leaf.

STRONG APEROL

Color of the cocktail: Orange
Servings: 1

ingredients
1 cl Amaretto
2 cl Aperol
1 cl brandy
1 shot of orange juice
150 ml sparkling wine
Ice cube

Preparation
Pour the ingredients into a long drink glass, top up with sparkling wine or mineral water, and serve with ice cubes if necessary.

ORANGE DUST

Color of the cocktail: Orange-brown
Servings: 1

ingredients
6 cl gin
6 cl hazelnut liqueur
12 cl coffee, cold brewed
1 orange slice
n. B.Tonic Water
Ice cube
possibly.coffee beans

Preparation
Cut a large slice from an orange. Pour half of it into a 0.5 l glass and squeeze it gently. Then add some ice cubes. Add the gin, liqueur and coffee and fill the glass with tonic water.

With the second orange slice, spread half of it once around the edge of the glass and then stick it to the glass as decoration. If you want to make the drink a little less sweet, you can add some coffee beans also fresh.

WATERMELON DAIQUIRI

Color of the cocktail: Pink
Servings: 4

ingredients
500 g watermelon, diced
10 cl rum, brown
2 tablespoons sugar, brown
6 cl lime juice or lemon juice
6 cl Triple Sec
Ice cubes or ice cubes

Preparation
Mix all ingredients in a blender to a smooth cocktail.
Divide into 4 glasses.

Of course, it also tastes good with fresh watermelon, but then the cocktail is more liquid and doesn't stay cool as long.

Quick and easy to prepare and a sweet summer cocktail.

CREAM COCKTAIL

Color of the cocktail: Pink
Servings: 4

ingredients
200 ml vodka
200 ml cream
250 ml raspberry syrup
250 ml vanilla yogurt
Ice cube

Preparation
Place all ingredients in a container and mix well.
Refrigerate and serve with ice cubes and drinking straw.

ADVOCAAT WITH SPARKLING WINE AND GRENADINE

Color of the cocktail: Pink
Servings: 1

ingredients
4 cl advocaat
2 cl Grenadine
Sparkling wine
2 ice cubes

Preparation
Put ice cubes into a glass and fill it halfway with a well-chilled sparkling wine. Stir in the advocaat and grenadine and then top up with sparkling wine.

STRAWBERRY KISS

Color of the cocktail: Pink-Orange
Servings: 1

ingredients
6 cl pineapple juice
10 cl orange juice
1 cl cream
50 ml sparkling wine
2 cl strawberry syrup
1 slice of lime
1 strawberry

Preparation
Shake the ingredients with 5-6 ice cubes in a shaker and strain into a long drink glass. Decorate with a slice of lime and strawberry.

TINTO DE VERANO

Color of the cocktail: Pink-Red
Servings: 1

ingredients
100 ml wine, rosé
200 ml lemonade
1 lime
1 lemon
Ice cube

Preparation
Gaseosa is a Spanish, slightly sweetened mineral water with a lemon taste. Alternatively, you could make your own Gaseosa from mineral water, with the juice of a lemon and a little sugar, or use a slightly sweetened lemon soda. Depending on how authentic you want it to be.

Place rosé wine and Gaseosa in the refrigerator hours before preparation and make ice cubes. Pour the ice cubes into a large glass. Mix the cooled rosé wine in a ratio of 1:2 with cooled Gaseosa. Cut the lime into slices and halve each slice. Put one slice of lime into each glass. Add a dash of lemon juice. The result is a refreshing summer drink that is very popular among Spaniards.

STRAWBERRY COLADA

Color of the cocktail: Pink-red
Servings: 2

ingredients
6 cl rum
10 cl pineapple juice
2 cl lemon juice
2 cl strawberry syrup
5 cl Cream of Coconut
Strawberries
Crushed ice

Preparation
Half fill a long drink glass with crushed ice. Mix all
ingredients and some strawberries with the electric
mixer, pour into the glass, and stir.

RAMAZZOTTI ROSATO DUO

Color of the cocktail: Rosé-Pink
Servings: 1

ingredients
5 cl liqueur (Ramazotti)
10 cl tonic water
Slices of lime
Ice cube

Preparation
Place the slices of lime in a wine glass and lightly toast.
Pour in Ramazzotti Aperitivo Rosato and Tonic Water
and add the ice cubes. Serve the aperitif with straw.

STRAWBERRY DAIQUIRI

Color of the cocktail: red
Servings: 1

ingredients
2 cl lime juice
5 cl rum, white
1 ½ Tbsp cane sugar, brown
6 strawberries
4 ice cubes
1 sprig of mint

Preparation
Place all ingredients in a blender and mix until
a homogenous drink is obtained.

Decorate with fresh mint.

9 PIN GIN

Color of the cocktail: red
Servings: 1

ingredients
4 cl gin
4 cl Lime Juice Cordial
2 cl lemon juice
2 cl currant syrup
4 ice cubes
10 cl mineral water
1 slice of lemon

Preparation
Put all ingredients into a glass of approx. 250 ml, stir, ready.

By adding mineral water, the taste can be individually
modified and adapted.

For the non-alcoholic version, simply leave out
the gin. Then it becomes the 9 pins free.

MAY TAI MIX

Color of the cocktail: red
Servings: 2

ingredients
2 cl rum, brown
2 cl rum, white
2 cl Amaretto
2 cl Triple Sec
2 cl almond syrup
2 cl cane sugar syrup
2 cl lime syrup
2 cl lime juice
200 ml multivitamin juice
2 cl Grenadine
8 ice cubes

Preparation

Place all ingredients in a cocktail shaker and pour vigorously for 20 seconds. You can also shake with some ice cubes. Then pour the Mai Tai into cocktail glasses and decorate with pineapple or other fruits.

LEMONADES LIQUEUR

Color of the cocktail: red
Servings: 1

ingredients
1 part Lillet
2 parts lemonade (e.g., Russian Wild Berry)
1 strawberry
5 ice cubes

Preparation
Pour Lillet into a wine glass, fill up with 4-5 ice cubes and pour Russian Wild Berry on top. Add quartered strawberry and stir carefully.

You can also use Tonic Water instead of Wild Berry. Then the cocktail is called Lillet Vive.

APEROL SPRAY

Color of the cocktail: red
Servings: 1

ingredients
3 cl Aperol
6 cl sparkling wine
1 shot of soda water
1 orange slice
Ice cube

Preparation
Place the orange slice in a large wine glass with a few ice cubes. Fill it up with Aperol, sparkling wine and soda and serve with a straw.

POMEGRANATE – SPARKLING WINE

Color of the cocktail: red
Servings: 2

ingredients
1 pomegranate
Mint leaves
300 ml sparkling wine
2 tsp grenadine

Preparation
Cut the pomegranate in half, then knock out the seeds or remove them with a spoon. Pour the seeds with mint leaves and the ice-cold sparkling wine into a jug and let it steep for 15 minutes. It is best to put them in the refrigerator.

Fish out the mint leaves and spread the grenadine syrup, the pomegranate seeds and the sparkling wine on two champagne glasses.

STRAWBERRY MOJITO

Color of the cocktail: red
Servings: 1

ingredients
2 hands strawberries
4 leaves mint
1 cl lime juice
2 teaspoons sugar, white
1 teaspoon sugar, brown
1 cl rum, white
Ice (ice cubes)
1 sprig of mint
Lemonade

Preparation
Puree 2 handfuls of strawberries and put them into a glass.
Add sugar, mint leaves and lime juice and mix well. Add the
Bacardi and fill the glass to about 1/3 with ice cubes. Fill
up with Sprite and garnish with the remaining mint.

It also tastes very delicious if you quarter a lime instead of the
strawberry puree, add the sugar and then crush it with a pestle.
The rest is done the same way as with the strawberry mojito.

TINTO DE VERANO

Color of the cocktail: red
Servings: 1

ingredients
100 ml wine, red
200 ml lemonade
2 cl wormwood
½ Sliced lime
3 ice cubes

Preparation
Pour all ingredients into a large glass, stir well and serve.

TOCCO ROSSO

Color of the cocktail: red
Servings: 1

ingredients
1 part Campari
1 part elderflower syrup
3 parts Prosecco
5 leaves mint

Preparation
Place all ingredients in a wine glass, add the fresh
mint leaves and stir carefully. Serve on ice.

APEROL LEMON SPRAY

Color of the cocktail: red
Servings: 1

ingredients
4 cl Aperol
150 ml bitter lemon
Ice cube
1 sprig of mint
Ginger, fresh

Preparation
Put some ice cubes in a wine glass, pour Aperol
over it and top up with Bitter Lemon.

Serve with a sprig of mint for even more freshness.
Press the mint in your hand a little to release
more aroma and pour into the glass.

If you like, you can also add a slice of fresh ginger.

STRAWBERRY - SPARKLING WINE

Color of the cocktail: red
Servings: 4

ingredients
70 g sugar
300 g strawberries
700 ml bottle of sparkling wine

Preparation
Mix strawberries, sugar and 300 ml. Then add the remaining 400 ml.

OUZO SPECIAL

Color of the cocktail: red
Servings: 1

ingredients
5 cl ouzo
200 ml lemonade
1 dash of grenadine
Ice cube

Preparation
You take a cocktail glass that holds at least 300 ml. Add 2-3 ice cubes (as desired), add the ouzo and top up with sprite. Finally add a dash of grenadine, which sinks to the bottom.

Serve with straw and enjoy hot summer days.

BEER COCKTAIL WITH GINGER ALE

Color of the cocktail: red
Servings: 1

ingredients
0.2 litre beer, light
0.1 litre ginger ale
1 cl Grenadine
1 dash of lemon juice
1 slice of lemon

Preparation

Pour the grenadine, lemon juice and ginger ale into a glass and mix. Pour the beer carefully so that it does not foam and put the lemon slice into the glass.

FRAGOLINO

Color of the cocktail: red
Servings: 2

ingredients
40 ml wild strawberry liqueur
200 ml prosecco, dry

Preparation
Spread the liqueur incl. fruits on two champagne
glasses and pour on Prosecco.

STRAWBERRY - LIME

Color of the cocktail: red
Servings: 1

ingredients
30 g strawberries
10 g sugar
6 ml lime juice
13 ml vodka
20 ml lemonade

Preparation
Wash the strawberries, mix them with all the liquid
ingredients and puree them with a blender.

Pass through a fine sieve and chill.

BICICLETTA - CAMPARI

Color of the cocktail: red
Servings: 1

ingredients
30 ml Campari
125 ml white wine, fruity, dry
1 dash of lime juice or lemon juice
Ice cube

Preparation
Pour the Campari into a glass. Add a dash of lime
juice or lemon juice and fill up with 1/8 litre of white
wine. Add ice cubes as desired and serve.

RASPBERRY MOJITO

Color of the cocktail: red
Servings: 2

ingredients
1 lime
4 teaspoons sugar
1 handful of raspberries
3 cl rum, white
2 sprigs of mint
Ice cube

Preparation
Cut the lime into eighths and divide into two glasses. Add
two teaspoons of sugar to each glass and squeeze the juice
from the limes with a pestle. Now squeeze a sprig of mint
a little bit per glass by hand so that the aroma can escape. I
twist the twigs and leaves until they tear open a little. Add
the raspberries, and if you like some ice cubes, fill up with
white rum and stir to distribute the sugar and lime juice.

If the raspberries were still too frozen, they did not
disintegrate by themselves, leave the drink to stand for
a while until the raspberries thaw and crush them with a
pestle or even a teaspoon until the drink turns red.

RHUBARB WINE

Color of the cocktail: red
Servings: 1

ingredients
100 ml rhubarb juice
100 ml white wine, dry
50 ml mineral water
1 strawberry

Preparation
Mix a spritzer from white wine and mineral water in a wine glass.
Add rhubarb juice and as a highlight add a strawberry.

On particularly hot days, frozen strawberries are particularly
suitable. The drink stays cool and is not diluted by ice cubes.

CAMPARI-O

Color of the cocktail: red
Servings: 1

ingredients
4 cl Campari
1 cl orange liqueur
8 cl grapefruit juice
5 cl wine, (Riesling)
1 piece orange
Ice

Preparation
Briefly shake the Campari with the liqueur and the juice with three ice cubes in a shaker. Pour into a long drink glass and top up with sparkling wine or Riesling. Put half an orange slice on the edge of the glass.

SPRITZ WITH ELDERBERRY AND BASIL

Color of the cocktail: red
Servings: 1

ingredients
2 cl Aperol
2 cl elderflower syrup
12 cl white wine
1 shot of sparkling mineral water
4 basil leaves
Ice cube

Preparation
Pour the aperol and elderflower syrup into the glass,
fill it up with wine and a shot of mineral water,
add basil leaves and ice cubes as desired.

COCKTAIL RUBY

Color of the cocktail: red
Servings: 1

ingredients
1 cl Grenadine
2 cl gin
10 cl grape juice, red
10 cl currant juice, black
Ice cube

Preparation
Put all ingredients together with some ice cubes in a cocktail shaker and shake well. Then pour everything into a wine glass and enjoy.

BLOODY CAIPIRINHA

Color of the cocktail: red
Servings: 1

ingredients
½ Lime
2 tsp cane sugar, brown
4 cl sugar cane schnapps
Ice cube
cherry juice
Grenadine

Preparation
Put the quartered lime and the cane sugar into a caipirinha
glass and crush it with a pestle. Add the caipirinha (if you like
it stronger, take 6 cl). Then fill the glass 3/4 with ice cubes and
add a shot of grenadine (depending on how sweet you like it).
Finally add some of the cherry juice until the glass is full.

STRAWBERRY - MARGARITA

Color of the cocktail: Red
Portions: 1

ingredients
100 g strawberries
25 ml tequila
15 ml orange liqueur
25 ml lemon juice
2 ice cubes

Preparation
Clean the strawberries, cut them into pieces and puree them finely. Put the puree in the freezer for about 3 hours.

Put the frozen strawberry puree together with the tequila, orange liqueur, lemon juice and ice cubes in a blender or mixer and mix everything thoroughly.

POMEGRANATE - DRINK

Color of the cocktail: red
Servings: 2

ingredients
2 pomegranates
Sugar
1 tsp lemon juice
150 ml sparkling wine

Preparation
Pre-cool the glasses.
Cut the pomegranates in half and set aside some seeds
for the garnish. Squeeze the juice and mix with sugar as
desired. Chill the squeezed juice for about 1 hour.
Just before serving, mix the pomegranate juice with the lemon
juice and pour it into the pre-cooled glasses. Top up with the
sparkling wine or mineral water. Garnish with the seeds set aside.

SHIRLEY

Color of the cocktail: red
Servings: 1

ingredients
1 part lemonade, white
1 part ginger ale
1 dash of grenadine
Ice cube

Preparation
Put ice cubes in a long drink glass. Pour white lemonade and ginger ale into the glass in equal parts. Add a dash of grenadine, stir and serve.

BEER SHOWER

Color of the cocktail: red
Servings: 1

ingredients
1 cl Grenadine
10 cl ginger ale
¼ Lime juice
Beer
Ice, crushed
1 cherry

Preparation
Fill a large glass 3/4 full with crushed ice. Add grenadine and ginger ale. Fill up with the alcohol-free beer and stir. Add cherry and lime as decoration on top.

RUM-COLA RED

Color of the cocktail: red
Servings: 1

ingredients
1 glass of cola
1 shot of currant juice
Ice cube
3 cl rum

Preparation
Mix everything and serve ice-cold.

SPICY APEROL

Color of the cocktail: red
Servings: 1

ingredients
3 cl Aperol
6 cl ginger beer
some ice cubes
1 sprig of rosemary
Cucumber slices
Olives

Preparation
Put the ice cubes in the glass. Pour Aperol over
them and fill up with ginger beer.
Add some cucumber slices as desired. A sprig of rosemary and 1
- 2 olives will also go well with the spiciness of the ginger berry.

CRANBERRY GIN & TONIC

Color of the cocktail: red
Servings: 1

ingredients
1 part gin
1 part cranberry juice
some ice cubes
1 piece of lemon
tonic water

Preparation
Pour the gin and cranberry juice into a glass and fill the glass to about 3/4 with ice cubes. Squeeze the piece of lemon into the glass and fill up with tonic water.

GRAPEFRUIT PALOMA

Color of the cocktail: red
Servings: 2

ingredients
2 tablespoons cane sugar
Lime juice
1 large grapefruit
6 cl tequila
n. B. Mineral water, well chilled
Ice cube

Preparation
Boil the cane sugar with 4 tablespoons of water and
let it cool down. Squeeze the grapefruit.
Fill 2 glasses with ice cubes. Mix the sugar syrup with grapefruit
juice and tequila and add a few squirts of lime juice.
Spread on the glasses and fill up with mineral water.

BORA - BORA

Color of the cocktail: red
Servings: 1

ingredients
6 cl passion fruit juice
10 cl pineapple juice
3 cl gin
2 cl lemon juice
1 cl Grenadine

Preparation
Mix all ingredients and pour into a glass.

SOWIK SUNRISE

Color of the cocktail: red
Servings: 1

ingredients
8 cl strawberry juice
2 kiwis
4 cl rum, brown
4 cl rum, white
2 cl lime juice
2 cl lemon juice
2 tablespoons of sugar
Ice

Preparation
Puree the kiwis with sugar, white rum, lime juice
and crushed ice in a mixer or hand blender.
Shake the strawberry juice with the brown
rum, lemon juice and ice in a shaker.
Pour the kiwi contents into a large glass, they should be
as thick as possible, if necessary put them into the freezer
beforehand. Carefully add the contents of the shaker.

GOOD NIGHT

Color of the cocktail: Red-brown
Servings: 1

ingredients
4 cl rum, brown
1 tablespoon honey syrup
¼ Organic lemon
120 ml lemonade
some ice cubes

Preparation
Pour rum and lemonade into a highball glass. Then stir the honey syrup in the glass until it has dissolved. Wash the lemon, quarter it, and pour it into the glass. Fill up with ice cubes.

SUMMER

Color of the cocktail: Red-orange
Servings: 1

ingredients
8 cl cherry juice
3 cl vodka
8 cl orange juice
6 cl banana nectar
2 cl vanilla syrup
some ice cubes

Preparation
Shake all ingredients together with ice in a shaker and pour into a cocktail glass with more ice cubes. If required, add a garnish to the glass, e.g., honeydew melon with cocktail cherry or apple wedge with physalis.

VODKA-CAMPARI-O

Color of the cocktail: Red-orange
Servings: 1

ingredients
3 cl vodka
1 cl Grenadine
3 cl Campari
5 cl orange juice
Ice cube

Preparation
Mix the ingredients in a long drink glass with some ice cubes.

GIN COCKTAIL

Color of the cocktail: White
Servings: 1

ingredients
1 part gin
2 parts lemonade
half orange
half lemon
half apple
¼ Cucumber
5 mint leaves

Preparation
Cut the orange, lemon, and cucumber into slices.
Core the apple and cut into slices. Put the mint leaves
together with fruit and cucumber in a large glass. Now
add the gin and fill up with lemonade as desired.

MOSCOW MULE

Color of the cocktail: white
Servings: 4

ingredients
16 cl vodka
800 ml ginger ale
½ Cucumber
1 sprig of mint
1 lime
Ice cube
Lime juice

Preparation
Peel the cucumber so that you get a stripe pattern. Or just leave it unpeeled and just wash it. Cut into slices or cut into eights lengthwise to make pencils (approx. 8-10 cm long). Fill glasses with ice cubes, fill each with 4 cl vodka and pour 200 ml ginger ale on each. Add 3-4 cucumber slices (or sticks) and a slice of lime. Garnish with mint or lemon balm. If you like, you can also add lime juice.

MOJITO

Color of the cocktail: White
Servings: 1

ingredients
4 pieces of lime
1 sprig of peppermint
1 tablespoon cane sugar, light
6 cl rum, white
6 ice cubes
30 cl mineral water

Preparation
Cane sugar with pieces of lime and a sprig of peppermint
glass and crush well. Add 6 cl white rum and mix. Put
4 ice cubes into the glass and stir. Fill up with mineral
water, stir briefly, and serve with a straw.

BASIL SMASH

Color of the cocktail: White
Servings: 1

ingredients
15 basil leaves
4 cl gin
2 cl lemon juice
2 cl sugar syrup, white
some ice cubes

Preparation
Put a few leaves of basil aside for decoration. Put the remaining ingredients together with some ice cubes into a cocktail shaker and shake very hard. Let it stand for a minute. This will give the Basil Smash a really nice green color.

Then pour the whole thing through a sieve onto new ice cubes, preferably in a tumbler. Decorate with basil leaves.

ELDERBERRY SPRITZER

Color of the cocktail: White
Servings: 1

ingredients
2 cl elderflower syrup
3 leaves mint
½ Lime
3 ice cubes
200 ml prosecco

Preparation
Pour the elderflower syrup into a glass and add 200 ml of cold
water or prosecco. Add mint, ice cubes and lime (cut into cubes).

RAFFAELLO - COCKTAIL

Color of the cocktail: White
Servings: 1

ingredients
4 cl vanilla flavored vodka
2 cl coconut rum
1 cl coconut syrup
1 cl almond syrup
5 cl cream
6 cl coconut milk
4 ice cubes

Preparation
Put all ingredients into the shaker, mix well, and pour into a long drink glass. Serve decorated with physalis and Raffaello.

GIN CHAMPAGNE

Color of the cocktail: white
Servings: 1

ingredients
Ice cube
45 ml gin
15 ml of lime juice
Champagne or dry sparkling wine
1 stem rosemary

Preparation
Mix ice cubes, gin, and lime juice in a bar shaker.
Strain through a bar strainer into a champagne or
champagne glass. Pour champagne or dry sparkling
wine and decorate with a sprig of rosemary.

COCONUT-BANANA MILK

Color of the cocktail: White
Servings: 2

ingredients
1 banana
400 ml of milk
8 cl Batida de Coco
Ice cube

Preparation
Puree the banana and mix with the remaining ingredients.
Fill two glasses with ice cubes.

GIN AND TONIC CUCUMBER

Color of the cocktail: White
Servings: 1

ingredients
4 cl gin
8 cl Tonic Water
2 slices of cucumber
3 ice cubes

Preparation
Together with 3 ice cubes, the cucumber slices are placed in a suitable glass jar. After that, deep-frozen gin is added and then the chilled tonic water.

TOM COLLINS

Color of the cocktail: White
Servings: 1

ingredients
5 cl gin
3 cl lemon juice
2 cl sugar syrup
Soda water
3 ice cubes

Preparation
Put the ice cubes into a chilled long drink glass. Put the first
3 ingredients on top and fill up with the soda water. Stir.

FROZEN GIN

Color of the cocktail: White
Servings: 1

ingredients
4 cl gin
2 cl lime juice
2 cl sugar syrup
120 ml bitter lemon

Preparation
Pour all ingredients into a highball glass. You can make your sugar syrup by mixing water and sugar 50:50 and heating it briefly.

MARTINI ROYALE

Color of the cocktail: White
Servings: 1

ingredients
5 cl wormwood
5 cl (Martini)
Ice cube
1 lime

Preparation
Fill a red wine glass with ice cubes. Squeeze the juice of half a lime over the glass.

Pour in the vermouth and sparkling wine in a ratio of 50/50 and add a piece of lime.

SUMMER SPRITZER

Color of the cocktail: White
Servings: 1

ingredients
¼ Lime
0,1-liter wine, white
0,1-liter tonic water
1 dash of lime syrup
2 ice cubes

Preparation
First, cut the lime quarter in half again, put it into a glass, and crush it. Then add the wine, tonic, and ice and refine with a dash of lime syrup. Then stir briefly.

SUN LIQUEUR

Color of the cocktail: white-beige
Servings: 1

ingredients
4 cl liqueur (Liqueur 43)
100 ml of milk
100 ml of orange juice
1 orange slice

Preparation
Mix everything in a nice tall glass with at least 250 ml capacity and decorate with the orange slice.

GIN FIZZ

Color of the cocktail: white-yellow
Servings: 1

ingredients
6 ice cubes
2 cl sugar syrup
4 cl gin
2 cl lemon juice
Mineral water

Preparation
Put the ice, gin, sugar syrup, and lemon juice into the shaker and shake briefly. Pour the whole into a long drink glass, add soda water until the glass is full and stir.

SPRAY LIMONCELLO

Color of the cocktail: white-yellow
Servings: 1

ingredients
4 cl limoncello
10 cl sparkling wine
5 cl bitter lemon
1 slice of lime
4 cl water
3 ice cubes

Preparation
Pour the limoncello into a champagne glass or long
drink glass and top up with the other ingredients.
Finally, serve with some ice cubes and a straw.

CODKA

Color of the cocktail: white-green
Servings: 1

ingredients
6 cl vodka
3 tsp cane sugar
2 cl lime juice
Lime pieces
Ice cube
1 slice of lime

Preparation
Pour the lime pieces into the glass. Add the cane
sugar and crush the lime pieces with a pestle.
Fill the glass with ice cubes, vodka, and lime juice.
Decorate the edge of the glass with a slice of lime.

IMPRINT OF THE PUBLISHER

Mindful Publishing

by

TTENTION Inc.
Wilmington - DE19806
Trolley Square 20c

Instagram: mindful_publishing
Contact: mindful.publishing@web.de